Infertility Can't Win!

One Woman's Journey to Motherhood

written by

Nashira Betton

Designed by JOSEP Book Designs (joseworkwork@gmail.com).

First Edition, 2019

ISBN 978-1-7335497-0-7

www.NashiraBetton.com

Infertility Protocol

Acknowledgements

Many, many thanks to:

My Lord & Savior Jesus Christ
Dr. Desiree McCarthy-Keith
Staff at Shady Grove Fertility (formerly Georgia Reproductive Specialists)
Ann-Marie Trimble
Jasmine Wilson-Holmes
Shanika Booth
Don Hardiman
Vanessa Hardiman
Logan Rena
Kendra Dee Photography
All the family and friends who supported me along my journey
&
Micah Betton

Prenatal Care

This book has been in the making for several years, and I'm super excited that you are able to share in this journey. It is also my hope that while reading this book, you will feel a sense of solidarity within the world of fertility and its many challenges.

The future of this book will be to create a series, providing real life stories of women and men facing infertility obstacles far and wide. Future editions will cover specific infertility challenges such as hormonal deficiencies, male factor, LGBT, cancer patients, etc. Your story should be read worldwide—imagine the impact it could have. To stay abreast of all future editions, subscribe via email at www.nashirabetton.com.

While reading, you'll notice that an email address, info@nashirabetton.com, has been noted at the end of each chapter. At some point, you may become inspired to share your story. I would love to develop a community where stories are shared, creating the encouragement needed to help us stay strong and resilient while we chase after our dream of parenthood.

At the end of each short chapter of this book, there are follow-up questions asked. These questions are there to help incite thoughts, memories, and details specific to you. However, you are not limited to sharing your story according to that format or the provoking questions. This is your world, so allow the creativity to flow. At the end of the book is an open space to capture your entire story but feel free to skip to typing, as that may come more natural to you.

Lastly, I'll ask for each of you to share, Share, SHARE the opportunity for others to tell their story. Just imagine if at the beginning of your journey, there had been a resource to read through, in which this awareness would've resulted in different, perhaps better, choices. Help to create a community for those fighting through infertility—let each one, teach one!

My heart is so fulfilled embarking upon this road, and I wish the same for you...

CHEERS!

FIRST
TRIMESTER

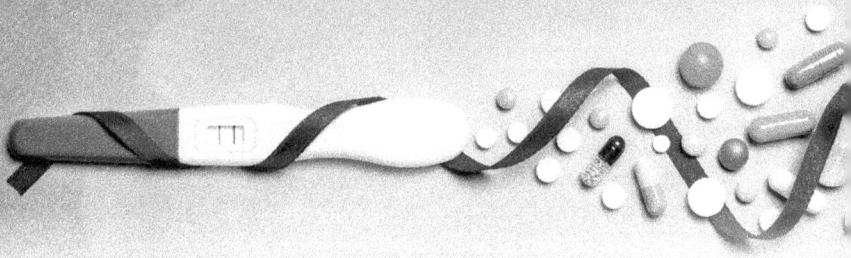

WHAT. DID. SHE. SAY?!

I always imagined that a part of my life would help the world by providing awareness to a cause and creating a community of support, but I never imagined it being by way of my hardest struggle yet my biggest victory.

As I began to write my story, I sat at my dining room table, 20 feet from my biggest victory, my biggest miracle, and the absolute love my life—my son.

The psychological distress, the emotional turmoil, and the physical pain to simply get to this point were all worth it. I'm here living the life that was custom made for me like a well-tailored suit on a Sunday morning.

Go grab a cup a tea (blame the Brit in me), a box of tissue,
and your favorite snuggle blanket as we have
some good ole' fashion infertility talk.
Cheers!

———— ·•◆◆•· ————

Just before my 22nd birthday in 2008, my OBGYN found a fibroid the size of a cantaloupe nestled inside of my uterus. It had attached itself to several sections of my uterine walls. It was far too large to have laparoscopic[1] surgery, so the only option was the invasive and quite scary, myomectomy[2] procedure.

I still remember it like it happened yesterday. I went into my OB's office doubled over, complaining of such painful cramps. I was all tears. The kind of cramps where you double, or even triple breathe, to gather just enough air to sob some more. My tears had shown to be too much for the worn through tissue I used. I could barely climb up on the examination table but I did, and straightaway assumed the fetal position. My doctor walked in and immediately grimaced. To see me like this gave her instant knowledge that something serious was going on.

She stretched me out as straight as she could to examine my pelvic area. I winced in pain but I knew I had no choice. As she pressed down on my abdomen, I clinched my teeth and balled up my fists as the pain was too much to simply not react in any way. She pressed around and let me know an internal and external sonogram was needed. Something didn't seem right.

Within a week, I was at a lab being examined by a sonogram technician. She told me absolutely nothing about what was displayed on the screen, no matter how many ways and times I asked. In retrospect, I'm glad she didn't. It wouldn't have ended well.

By the next week, I received the results in the mail and a directive to follow-up with my OB—you know the doctor

---

[1] Laparoscopic - is a surgical procedure that involves making one, two, or three very small cuts in the abdomen, through which the doctor inserts a laparoscope and specialized surgical instruments.

[2] Myomectomy – surgical procedure to remove uterine fibroids

all of us ladies have a love-hate relationship with. Now, listen. The results had a bunch of jibber-jabber and numbers followed by centimeters. I don't know about you but I'm an inches kind of gal and none of it made relative sense. I now realize that's because I wasn't expecting anything alarming.

Days later, here I am back in my OB's office across the desk from her, while she's holding the same rubbish I received in the mail. As impatient as I am (because I am) I asked her to get to the bottom line. She proceeded to tell me that I have a tumor the size of a cantaloupe that needed to be removed via a bikini line incision. Within seconds, I was hyperventilating into uncontrollable tears!

What. Did. She. Say?!
(All I heard was tumor and being sliced & diced)

Fast forward: during the winter break of 2008, I was met with a successful surgery. The bikini line cut was ugly but hey, at least I was tumor free. The tumor was benign—thank the heavens! However, she did say that I would never be able to have a natural delivery and that I may experience challenges getting pregnant. She was more clairvoyant than she knew but honestly, I was 22 and the last thing on my mind was getting knocked up so who cared, right?! Right.

Stats

ICI unsuccessful attempts = 2
Total Cost = $2600

Have you had an OBGYN scare long before you were even thinking about getting pregnant?

_____

_____

_____

What surgeries, if any, have you had during your journey?

_____

_____

_____

Have there been procedures, if done earlier in your life that would have made you successful [sooner]?

_____

_____

_____

Share your story at info@nashirabetton.com ♥

_____ ⋅⋅◆◆◆⋅⋅ _____

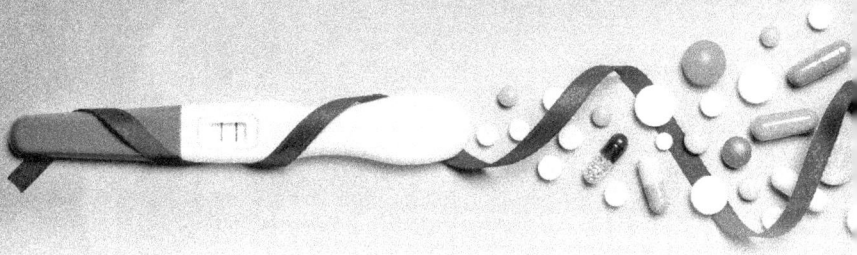

CUPID STRUCK ME

Summer 2012, I was a single woman living in the nation's capital, in the peak of my career and loving life. Then, it hit me. Cupid struck me with the baby fever arrow. The strike was like labor pains—intense but well worth it. Loads of thoughts came rushing at one time but I sifted to the most important facts: I had a tumor removed from my uterus 4 years before and still suffered from the monthly anguish of endometriosis[3]. How in the hell was I going to have a baby? Like, REALLY have a baby! Fearlessly, I started down my very own personalized, hell-riddled path to motherhood.

I figured there had to be a way to get pregnant via turkey basting. Let me be honest: I had not met the love of my life and I wasn't going to waste any more time waiting. I found a few websites and YouTube pages that spelled out how to get the job done. I was all set to go (or so I thought). How naïve of me.

Once I believed I was equipped with the right knowledge, I went to the store and purchased ovulation sticks, pre-seed, and menstrual cups for my upcoming activities. For the next

---

[3]   Endometriosis - is a condition where the lining of the uterus grows outside of the uterus. It is an abnormal and often painful disorder that affects anywhere from six to 10 percent of women.

week or so, I spent every morning testing for ovulation by awaiting my LH surge[4]. In parallel, I received the proper authorization from my OB/GYN to pick-up sperm from a cryobank just 20 miles south of where I lived.

I'd be lying if I don't say I was anxious. I was nervously excited as I had continuous daydreams about the sperm meeting the egg then commencing with a tango. I was equally excited that I would be able to brag to the world that I got my own self pregnant in the comfort of my bedroom!

One Thursday morning when the sticks detected my soon-to-happen ovulation, I hopped in my car. Off I went, on my journey to pick up my paid purchase of Donor #12345's sperm to turkey baste (also known as Intracervical Insemination[5]) that evening. I followed all the directions I'd gathered through my research down to the letter. Oven mitts in hand. I removed the two vials of sperm, poured them into the menstrual cup, and inserted it carefully. Propped my butt up on a few pillows and envisioned the sperm meeting the egg during the horrid two-week wait[6].

The next couple weeks were awful and the first of many more emotional rollercoasters. I symptom spotted out of control. It was ridiculous and so was I! I remember my left eye jumping after an eyelash fell out and you could not

[4]   Luteinizing Hormone (LH) Surge – it triggers the start of ovulation, and the most fertile period of the menstrual cycle occurs.

[5]   Intracervical Insemination (ICI) - involves placing sperm directly into the woman's reproductive tract to improve the chances of pregnancy.

[6]   Two Week Wait - time it takes a fertilized egg implants in the uterine wall to start emitting enough of the hCG hormone to be detected by the beta blood pregnancy test.

make me believe that wasn't a sign from the universe. Ha! Silly rabbit.

As I approached the end of my two-week wait, the only symptom I could feel was devastation. The feeling of defeat as my cycle started, the accompanying pain, and the realization that I was not with child. What did I do wrong? How did I mess up this easy process? Am I really out of the $1300 I spent on those 2 measly vials of sperm?

ICI #1: Unsuccessful

This cannot be real.

After I gathered myself and finished wallowing in self-pity, I decided I was going to try again. Let's face it, I'm a typical Type-A personality, and the perfectionist in me could not be okay with failure.

I started sharing my baby aspirations with friends who had kids just so I wouldn't feel so alone. Lo and behold, one of my friends had her son, let's call him 'M', by turkey basting at-home on her couch. She explained to me the details of her method (identical to every article read and video watched), where she purchased sperm, and how she coped during the two-week wait. To top it all off, 'M' was conceived during my friend's first and only try with ICI!

Now, armored with a positive anecdote and within my next ovulation window, I knew without a shadow of a doubt that I had gotten all of the steps to turkey basting accurate. I was very confident that I had gotten it right. I even made a tutorial video on <u>YouTube</u>, helping countless other women get pregnant. Just like that, with two more vials and weeks later I was met with the dreaded Aunt Flow.

ICI #2: Unsuccessful

Again, what did I do wrong? Why wasn't this working for me but other women achieved success? I was so bewildered with thoughts of other women's success, but there was me: deserving, capable, and willing yet I could not figure this sh*t out!

So, I quit.

Wallowing in the crescendo of self-pity, only after try number two—boy, did I have a long way to go—I gave up! I resolved that the Universe didn't want me to have kids so I just wouldn't. Completely irrational and extreme, I decided that this very moment was the end of my road for motherhood. Screw it!

Stats

ICI unsuccessful attempts = 2
Total Cost = $2600

When were you when cupid struck you
with the baby fever arrow?

_____

_____

_____

How did you let failure stop you on your journey?

_____

_____

_____

How have you coped with the thoughts
of other parents' success?

_____

_____

_____

Share your story at info@nashirabetton.com ♥

——————— ✦✦✦✦✦✦ ———————

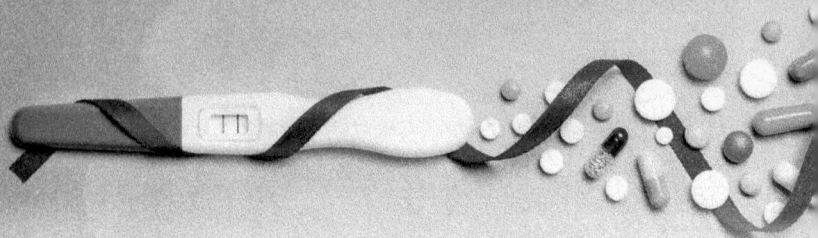

SHE CALLED!

Social media has connected me to so many people far and wide, and for that, I am eternally grateful. Instagram is such a powerful tool, and it gave me my first glimpse of hope to motherhood.

I had been following on Instagram[7], a young lady who had conceived her beautiful daughter via intrauterine insemination (IUI)[8] on the first try. She posted baby pictures of her donor, baby pictures of herself, and baby pictures of her IUI conceived daughter. I was so riddled with emotion, I did the only thing a sane person would do. I wrote my phone number under a picture from 83 weeks before (this was before direct message existed), politely demanded she call me because I had questions that needed immediate answers!

There you have it folks; the Universe sent me my Hail Mary after declaring that I quit this journey the year before. Again, you could not tell me that I had not found the solution to all my problems. There's the extremist showing her ugly head, again.

---

[7]   Instagram – a photo and video-sharing social networking service.

[8]   IUI - the procedure itself involves transferring specially washed semen directly into the uterus via a thin catheter.

She responded to my 83-week old post and I nearly peed myself. The anxiety was real. I mean, you would have thought she was writing me a check for 1 billion dollars, or at least that is what it felt like. She told me she would call on her break and I nearly had heart failure. I was GLUED to my phone awaiting her call.

She called, guys. SHE CALLED!

I could barely run out of my office fast enough to take this highly anticipated and highly classified (because of course, it had to be top-secret) phone call. I walked laps around the office complex and learned everything I could about having a baby.

As you can tell, I was no longer quitting my motherhood journey or at least, just not right now.

We talked for well over an hour, and I bled her for all the information I could get: from cryobank information to her specific doctor to all the details on the medication. The only catch was that she resided in Atlanta, Georgia and I lived in Washington, DC. How in the world was I going to make use of all this good information AND get pregnant from 700 miles away?

I had a full tank of gas, vacation days, a birthday to celebrate, and determination that wouldn't let me give up. Two months later in November, during Fall 2012, I was driving down to Atlanta to have my first round of IUIs done by the Instagram mom's fertility doctor. Dr. H had ordered fertility medication that I began to take before getting to Atlanta as well as set up all of the necessary appointments for monitoring and the actual insemination.

On my birthday and 6 mature follicles later, I was inseminated—Happy Birthday to me... or not!

IUI Attempt #1: Unsuccessful

<u>Stats</u>

ICI unsuccessful attempts = 2
IUI unsuccessful attempts = 1
Total Cost = $4750

*How has social media helped or hindered
you with your process?*

_____

_____

_____

What is the craziest thing you've done to become pregnant?

_____

_____

_____

*Did you have a person you looked to for
guidance during your journey?*

_____

_____

_____

Share your story at info@nashirabetton.com ♥

⋅⋅◆◆◆◆⋅⋅

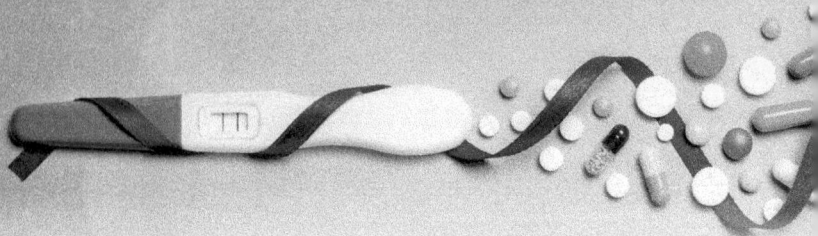

WHY DIDN'T ANYONE STOP ME?!

Right before the Christmas holiday season, I found myself without child and in the deepest depression I could imagine, at the time. I was not pregnant and at my wits end. I just could not understand why it didn't work and what to do next. I felt hopeless and like a horrible joke was being played on me but no one was laughing.

The worst part was that I made the mistake of telling my closest friends and family. They knew I had been trying to get pregnant and were also emotionally attached and excited for me to conceive a child. So, I had to deal with their disappointment, too. It felt draining to coddle them and myself at the same time. It was all too much for me to handle. I then sank into depression.

In hindsight, I was oscillating between three of the five stages of loss and suffering. I was completely out-of-order. I was in, what felt like, an infinite loop of anger-bargaining-depression or any permutation thereof, and did not see a way out. I dwelled in bargaining and depression a lot but every now and again, I'd sprinkle some anger in there to round it out. I was losing my mind and could not escape my very own infertility purgatory.

So I did what any headstrong woman—this wasn't going to beat me—desiring motherhood would do. In less than a month, I semi-fine-tuned a half-baked plan. I found some ducks and put them in a row. I packed up every morsel of my belongings and relocated to Atlanta to aggressively follow my pursuits to becoming a mum!

When I think back to this moment in my journey, so many thoughts and questions come to mind, making me laugh hysterically. First and foremost, what kind of deductive reasoning was I using that allowed me to conclude moving over 700 miles was the smartest thing to do?! How was I so confident that my job would allow me to work remotely? Why didn't anyone stop me?! But above all else, was there no other doctor in my immediate metropolitan area that could've gotten me to the same exact finish line with less hassle? And funny enough, I still don't have answers to these questions…

But I can tell you one thing, I was a woman with a mission and planned to be unstoppable!

Stats

ICI unsuccessful attempts = 2
IUI unsuccessful attempts = 1
Total Cost = $4750

How have you handled being childless during holidays?

_____

_____

_____

*Who are some of the people you comforted
during your failed attempt(s)?*

_____

_____

_____

*What are some things you've done in your
journey you can laugh at today?*

_____

_____

_____

Share your story at info@nashirabetton.com ♥

————— ‹‹♦♦♦›› —————

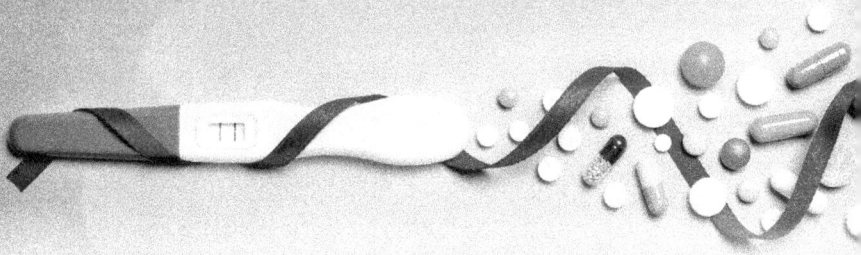

THIS TIME

Twelve hours later with a loaded truck and car hitched on a trailer, I arrived to my final destination of Atlanta, Georgia in Spring 2013 with my eyes on the baby dust prize. I was able to find a cozy apartment in North Atlanta where I immediately became settled and back on my baby making journey.

Having lived in Atlanta before, I quickly became reacquainted with my network but most importantly, I began developing mummy friends I could leverage as support. With this new found support and all the courage I could muster up, I was back to scheduling appointments with Dr. H's office for IUI round #2.

This time, I felt better prepared. This time, I wasn't pressured by limited vacation days. This time, there wasn't stress on my body from driving hundreds of miles. This time, I didn't have the anxiety of timing ovulation perfectly. This time, I lived 15 minutes from the doctor's office. This time, my appointments were set to really accommodate my schedule. This time, my prescriptions were filled by my doctor's pharmacy. This time, it was foolproof.

This time, the dosage of my Clomid [9] mediation had been increased. This time, I had created SIX strong and viable eggs. This time, I gave myself the trigger shot[10] like a 3rd year medical student. This time, I planned and completed TWO inseminations: one right before ovulation and one right after. This, time the two-week wait felt like a vacation on the beach. This time, it was so easy and so perfect just the way it should be...

...and this time, I got a Big. Fat. Negative[11].

IUI Attempt #2 and #3: Unsuccessful

I was mortified. I just wanted to die. I wanted baby Jesus in the manger to scoop me up and take me to the afterlife. I had had enough.

Everything was perfect! WTF happened?! How could it not work again, especially when this go around happened flawlessly? Why does my body hate me so much? What could I have done differently? What should the doctor have done differently? Why isn't this working? Why did I feel pregnant but actually wasn't? Why can't I get this right?

I was so angry with my body, my doctor, and God. I cursed them all. Yes, each and every showstopper I cursed. I did so until I felt I reached the level of justification for such

---

[9]   Clomid - ovulatory stimulating drug used to help women who have problems with ovulation.

[10]   Trigger Shot - is a medication used after other fertility hormones to induce ovulation (release of the egg from the ovary) or to induce final maturation of the egg(s).

[11]   Big Fat Negative - negative pregnancy test

self-hate, misguided out lashing, and flat-out blasphemy. Spawned out of anger and the feeling of defeat, I schedule my appointments for IUI #4.

I'm so glad I can now look back at this journey and smile.

Stats

ICI unsuccessful attempts = 2
IUI unsuccessful attempts = 3
Total Cost = $9050

Did you create support networks during your journey?

_____

_____

_____

How have you dealt with the two-week wait?

_____

_____

_____

*What are some of the emotional rollercoasters
you've experienced during the journey?*

_____

_____

_____

Share your story at info@nashirabetton.com ♥

SECOND
TRIMESTER

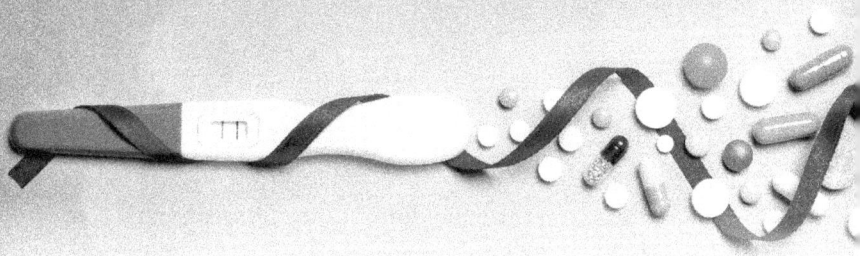

FIVE TWENTY SEVEN

With round #4, I was going to do things slightly different by being more assertive. I decided to actually have a true consultation with the doctor and asked probing questions until I felt we were better equipped for the next round. The end result of my consultation produced doctor's orders for bloodwork. The same bloodwork that had never been done before. This is where my suspicions set in.

Why on earth had I never been informed, suggested, or demanded to have blood drawn before? Why wasn't this a part of the round #2/#3 regimen? If I hadn't probed, would we have skipped blood work this round too? So now I'm angry, again.

Admittedly, I never did ask these questions to the doctor because with my inductive reasoning, I concluded this doctor was money hungry and the answers wouldn't have changed anything. At this point, including round #2/#3, I was 2 ICI tries, 3 IUI procedures, and 7 vials of semen in the hole. For those of you who like numbers, that's ~$4500 (3 IUI) + ~$4550 (7 vials) = ~$9050 of cold cash paid to the motherhood process.

Although I knew I should've been grateful because my health insurance did cover my diagnostic testing and some fertility medication, I was still pissed that I had nothing to show for all that I had been through up to latest rounds. Filled with rage, I then questioned the doctor on the purpose of every drop of blood taken, the change in medication to Femara[12] after the blood draw, and the precise timing designated for the insemination.

As a result, I became knowledgeable about my egg quality[13], follicle stimulation hormone (FSH[14]), luteinizing hormone (LH), estradiol hormone (E2[15]), anti-mullerian hormone (AMH[16]), and the list goes on. But most importantly, I learned that I could grow eggs but on Clomid, the quality wasn't the greatest. So Femara was my prescribed drug.

As the idiom suggests, knowledge is power, and I was soundly equipped to receive my BFP[17].

Throughout round #4, I took my medications on time, we monitored my egg growth meticulously, and we prepared for a great insemination post LH surge. The day of my insemination felt like the stars were aligning for me. I showed up to my insemination appointment 30 minutes ahead of time just to be on the safe side. I signed in at the

---

[12] Femara - fertility medication prescribed for women experiencing ovulation problems and/or unexplained infertility

[13] Egg Quality – refers to the state of an egg as genetically normal or abnormal.

[14] FSH – hormone that can directly influence your chances of conceiving and/or sustaining pregnancy.

[15] E2 – determines your ovaries' ability to produces eggs.

[16] AMH – protein hormone produced by special cells inside the ovarian follicles.

[17] BFP (Big Fat Positive) – positive pregnancy test.

receptionist desk and impatiently waited for my turn to jump on the heavenly, stork guided insemination table.

As my appointment time approached, I became concerned. Concerned because my doctor wasn't in the office yet. Anxious ole' me politely asked the receptionist where Dr. H was and if we were still on for my 3:30 insemination. From that I found out he had a day full of surgeries. Now y'all, God bless the women he was surgically working on but this was my time to shine so being tardy for the insemination party was NOT going to work, for obvious reasons.

At my appointment time, I inquired with the receptionist to speak with the head nurse on staff. Speaking with the head nurse, she assured me that he would be on his way soon. I learned his last surgery ran over time, but since the doctor's office adjoined to the local hospital, he'd be over in a flash.

I was hot. I was fuming. I couldn't believe this was happening to me but there was nothing I could do. I decided to harness my chi and chill out. It was now 3:50pm, which quickly turned to 4:15pm then magically turned to 4:55pm. It was FIVE TWENTY SEVEN post meridiem when Dr. H finally came through the doors. I was fighting back tears as I journeyed back to the fiery hell, demon-guided insemination table.

Anyone who has been through this process knows that for every minute sperm is not in your uterus waiting to meet its beloved egg, is every minute that egg could be disintegrating into AF's[18] black hole.

---

[18]   AF (Aunt Flow) - a popular euphemism referring to the menstrual cycle.

I laid there on the table in premeditated conquest. There was no hope to garner. I knew we had missed our window of opportunity.

And I was right.

IUI Attempt #4: Unsuccessful

One thing I was really proud of myself for, as a lesson learned this time, I did not tell anyone I had been going through the process again. On the upside, I didn't have to console anyone when these rounds did not work, but on the downside, I had no one to soothe me.

Stats

ICI attempts = 2
IUI attempts = 4
Total Cost = $11200

How early in the process did you have bloodwork done?

_____

_____

_____

*What medications have you used
throughout your infertility journey?*

_____

_____

_____

What money concerns have you experienced with this process?

_____

_____

_____

Share your story at info@nashirabetton.com ♥

◆◆◆◆◆◆

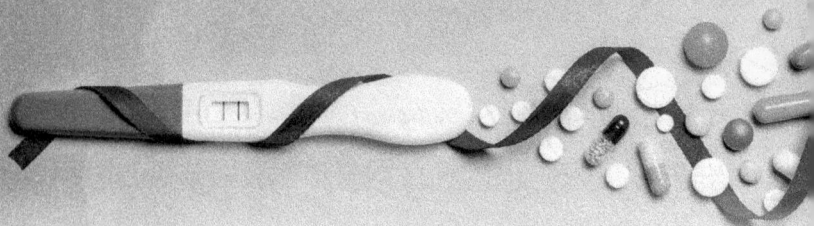

GUTTED X 2!

Needless to say I fired that doctor.

At this point, I knew I had to move on to a new practice and a new doctor. After doing some cursory research, because at this point impatience set in, I found a Reproductive Center that appeared to fit my needs. I had to wait two weeks for my consult, but I figured I'd come this far so what was another 2 weeks.

During my dreaded two week wait (the irony…ha!) for my consultation appointment, the fertility center hosted an evening seminar with a panel consisting of one of their RE doctors and a pregnant patient with a success story. I thought to myself, "this is exactly what you need to move the dial in the right direction."

As that evening approached, I was filled with such assurance that this was the precursor to my gold at the end of my rainbow. In true fashion, I showed up early and stayed late to ask every question I could think of. The doctor was very knowledgeable and really had a passion for his practice but admittedly, I wasn't so interested in what he had to say. I wanted to hear all about the success story from their patient since that's the seat I so longed to sit in.

She told the story of her and her husband trying for years to no avail. She mentioned all the tests she and her husband had done, which is where she found out that her egg quality had deteriorated to nothing.

I was gutted x 2!

I'll be honest, I felt bad for her. Even though she was clearly pregnant, I knew what her fate meant: donor eggs. But selfishly, I also knew that her fate meant she had to go through IVF[19], the very process I was trying to avoid at all cost. Her success story was inspiring, but also deflating. That wasn't the narrative I was expecting to hear that evening.

I stayed after and asked a plethora of questions to learn more about the intricacies of her process. I had hoped to hear about IUIs and her challenges with that—but there were none. You might ask, "Why would you want to hear about her IUI challenges?" The hyper-analytical side of me wanted to have a story to compare mine to and pick a part where she went "wrong" with hopes of finding the lynchpin for my success.

She provided me encouraging words and even gave me her number to stay in touch. She also stated that *if I had to go through IVF,* she would give me all of her leftover medication, which would save me loads of money. I left the seminar wiser and ready to ask all the right questions this time.

Excited and ready to get this show on the road, I showed up to my morning consultation appointment 30 minutes

---

[19]   IVF (In Vitro Fertilization) - the process of fertilization by extracting eggs, retrieving a sperm sample, and then manually combining an egg and sperm in a laboratory dish. The embryo(s) is then transferred to the uterus.

early. As I waited in the sitting room, I saw so many smiling faces and just knew I was at the right spot. Keeping with my trend, I impatiently sat and counted down the minutes on the clock.

It was finally my turn and I was escorted back to my new RE's office. To my surprise and excitement, my new doctor was the RE from the seminar I attended. A sigh of relief came over me. I told him all about my previous attempts and haphazard processes I experienced. I let him know that I was willing to do whatever it took to get me to a success story.

His next comment made me see red. Based on what he heard, he without a shadow of a doubt felt that IVF was my only way to get the baby I so desperately wanted. He said he had his team's Financial Advisor ready to speak with me and in she walked as he walked out. She showed me a packet of information and inundated me with pricing, embryo testing options, timing, etc.

I was overwhelmed. I thanked her for her time and walked out.

As I drove down the highway frustrated and confused, I couldn't for the life of me understand how the doctor had determined so quickly and without testing that I needed to proceed with IVF. I know I told him all about my previous attempts, but something didn't add up to me. It felt like he was prepared to tell me IVF was the main course meal no matter what story I had for him. He had the IVF Financial Advisor on standby for goodness sake!

It was more than clear to me using that Fertility Center was not an option.

Stats

Still…
ICI attempts = 2
IUI attempts = 4
Total Cost = $11200

*Did you experience switching practices
during your journey? If so, why?*

_____

_____

_____

Have you attended seminars and were they helpful?

_____

_____

_____

*Have you ever felt like a doctor or
practice was on a money grab?*

_____

_____

_____

Share your story at info@nashirabetton.com ♥

————— ✦✦✦✦✦ —————

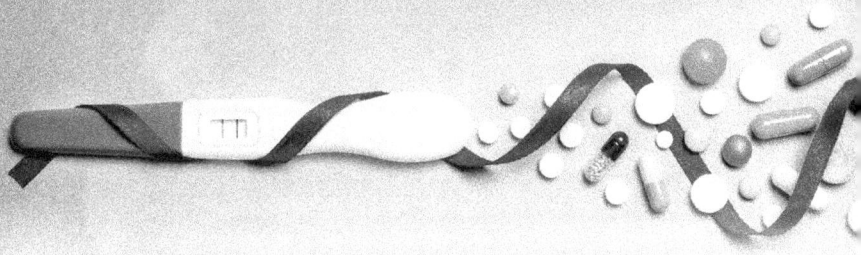

CHATTANOOGA, TENNESSEE

In my younger years, desperation for me resulted in really chaotic logic (I own my "crazy" *haha*). My newfound logic: throw the entire state of Georgia's Reproductive Endocrinologists away—right in the trash. So that's just what I did. I pursued REs in a bordering state—Tennessee.

Based on recommendations of my insurance company, in the beginning of 2014, I selected the first practice within a reasonable drive. I reached out to the practice to set up my consultation appointment, and I did so with little to no zeal; we know how much I love consultation appointments and how great they turned out for me previously.

On the day of my consultation appointment, I set out on a 2 ½ hour drive to Chattanooga, Tennessee from Atlanta, Georgia. I was their first appointment of the day, so I didn't get the opportunity to see any smiling faces, but that theory had clearly been dispelled with the last experience. However, I did enjoy the ambiance of the Tennessee Infertility practice, so I found internal comfort and nested there.

I was led back to Dr. S' office where I explained the entire rundown of my infertility journey and my desires from the process moving forward. I explained to her that I wanted to be well educated and informed about every step she was going to recommend I adhere to. I told her about the two practices and experiences I encountered, and wanted to be sure that those situations wouldn't be repeated here. Dr. S encouragingly asked what I wanted to do next and I told her: an IUI with perfect timing. She obliged.

Pumped up and ready for my next perfect IUI, I headed home and began proper preparation for IUI #5.

First, I reached out to my preferred cryobank to place an order for two vials of my favorite donor's sperm, because (duh!) that's most important. Then, I called my insurance company to confirm portions of the medication cost would be covered. Lastly, I ravenously and copiously ate as much pineapple core as possible *haha*. Pineapple contains bromelain, which is said to help with implantation[20] since it has anti-inflammatory capabilities. This is important as you want the embryo[21] to nestle itself in the uterus like a homebuyer in a new home.

We embarked upon the proper routine: scheduled appointment, conducted bloodwork, submitted prescriptions, and on two peak ovulation days, I was inseminated within 36 hours of each other…

IUI Attempt #5 and #6: Unsuccessful

Again, I was met with failure.

The major difference in my thought process regarding this disappointing cycle lies in my belief that Dr. S actually

---

[20] Implantation - the process of the egg burrowing into the uterine lining of the uterus

[21] Embryo - an unborn offspring in the process of development.

did everything right and it just wasn't my turn to meet victory. Also, she stated that as she inflated my uterus for insemination, she felt something "abnormal" and wanted to investigate it more as a possible reason for the failure. It was now my turn to oblige.

Stats

ICI attempts = 2
IUI attempts = 6
Total Cost = $15500

What crazy logic have you held strong to during the process?

_____

_____

_____

Did you ever officially nest with your RE practice?

_____

_____

_____

*How did you maintain your confidence in
your RE and their recommendations?*

_____

_____

_____

Share your story at info@nashirabetton.com ♥

———— ++++++ ————

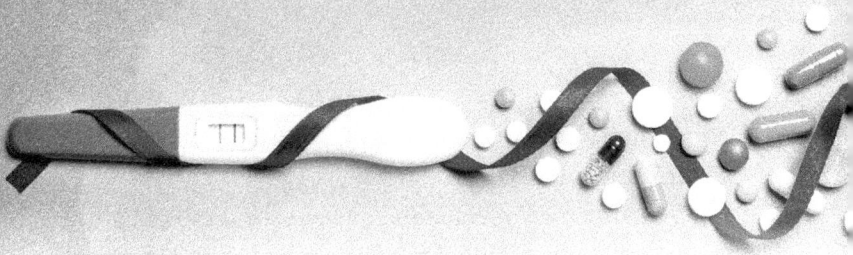

SOUND FAMILIAR?

Looking back, I'm grateful the last IUIs didn't work despite the disappointment and money down the drain. Had it worked more avoidable problems would've been endured.

Dr. S. ordered an internal and external sonogram (*sound familiar?*) to take a closer look at what she thought she felt during the insemination. Within 2 weeks of the failed IUI, we conducted the sonogram and her suspicions were correct. I had, again, grown fibroid tumors. The added cherry on top were the, also growing, cysts.

As Dr. S described what she saw during the sonogram, I knew that automatically meant surgery of some sort, I just didn't know how invasive. She saw a number of fibroids, a few cysts, and some scar tissue from the surgery I had 6 years prior. Luckily, she did say the removal of these obstructions would not require me being cut wide open but instead outpatient laparoscopic surgery would suffice.

Once the exam was completed, I worked with the local Chattanooga hospital to get my surgery date scheduled. I also mentally prepared for success.

Success is what I wanted, and success is what I received.

The surgery went well, and every obstruction was removed. Since it was an outpatient surgery and my recovery was minimal, we were able to go right into my next IUI cycle. Bring it on IUI #7 and #8!!

Y'all, I know I'm crazy and move at the speed of light. I think back to the details of this journey and realize I brought a lot of misery to myself because of my complete impatience. But as nature would have it, I was chasing down an egg, and nothing was going to stop or delay the gratification I was seeking.

I, yet again: ordered 2 vials, confirmed medication coverage, and ate as many pineapples as possible. This was the time it was going to work! This time, we removed ALL potential challenges. This time, we had the right formula. This time we inseminated 30-hours apart. This time, we were better prepared. This time, we were…

IUI Attempt #7 and #8: Unsuccessful

WTF?! I was in disbelief, and the doctor was too.

To her, this was the picture-perfect cycle. My follicles looked great, I triggered and inseminated on time, and there weren't any complications keeping this from working. She wanted to investigate further because something wasn't adding up to her. But what was adding up, for me, were all the costs: ~$12000 ($1500 x 8 IUIs) + ~$7800 (12 vials) = ~$19800!

Stats

ICI attempts = 2
IUI attempts = 8
Total Cost = $19800

*Have you ever experience a moment of
de'ja' vu during this process?*

_____

_____

_____

*Did you ever have a picture-perfect cycle?
What was your experience?*

_____

_____

_____

*Did you keep track of the costs during your
journey? If so, how much was spent?*

_____

_____

_____

Share your story at info@nashirabetton.com ♥

⋅⋅⋅♦♦♦⋅⋅⋅

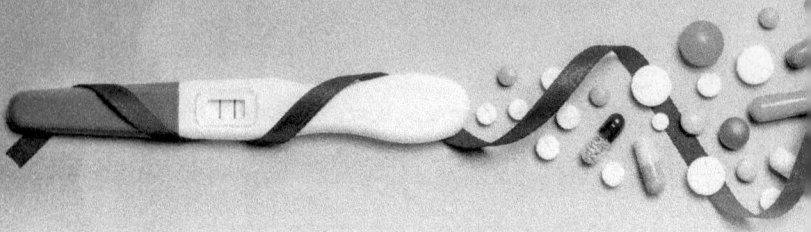

FACE PALM

Dr. S' final recommendation was to get a holistic view of my uterus and everything in that cavity with a dye test[22]. Unaware of what a dye test meant, I immediately thought it was another surgery—silly me. But it did require me to schedule the procedure with a special facility.

Anyone that has taken a dye test knows how uncomfortable it is. Between what feel likes someone jamming a straw into your cervix and the actual dye that is pumped into your uterine cavity, I just knew I was going to walk toward the light. The pain I felt was indescribable. To make matters worse, I had to stay as still as possible for x-ray photos and videos to be taken while dye was injected.

The test was finally over, and I had to [im]patiently wait for the facility to provide my RE with the recordings.

Within the next couple of weeks, I was back in the Dr. S' office to hear about the results and her conclusions from the dye test. She had previously viewed the results of the recordings on her own but gave me the opportunity to view it with her again. As we watched the video and looked at the

---

22   Dye Test (HSG) - It involves placing an iodine-based dye through the cervix and taking x-rays to help evaluate the shape of the uterus and whether the fallopian tubes are blocked

images, she explained exactly what was happening and why. By the end of the last image, I understood that my fallopian tubes function abnormally and rest fully open.

Normal fallopian tubes contract open and shut. This process aides the egg in moving down toward the uterus after it's released from the follicle attached to the ovary. In theory, the sperm swims through the cervix and waits until it meets the egg in the uterus. Voila, magic happens.

Women who suffer from my particular abnormality run a risk of an ectopic[23] pregnancy, which is never good in the grand scheme of things. It was concluded that it was a blessing in disguise that I had never gotten pregnant because it would have likely occurred in my fallopian tube(s), resulting in surgery. But this also meant the likeliness of IUIs working for me was slim to none.

I didn't want to feel robbed of the opportunity to become pregnant in the seemingly, easiest way. I didn't want to believe IUI wouldn't work for me, so I didn't. In my own gluttony for punishment, I tried again *face palm*.

This IUI cycle I had convinced myself that maybe the donor was a problem too. To clear any bad energy, I switched cryobanks and donors to ensure optimal success. And I'm glad I did! While learning so much about the process of getting pregnant, I hadn't done much research on sperm in general. After digging deep into Dr. Google, I learned about Cytomegalovirus[24] also known as CMV.

Admittedly, I should've learned about this long before trying to get pregnant but everything happens as it's

---

[23]   Ectopic - an unborn offspring in the process of development.

[24]   Cytomegalovirus - – is a member of the herpes family of viruses that also includes chickenpox and mono.

supposed to. CMV when passed to a child can result in hearing or vision loss, disability, seizures, etc. For these reasons, it is important to avoid procreating with someone who is a carrier of the virus, if you can help it. In my case, I could help it so I did moving forward. In hindsight, I'm grateful that none of the previous attempts worked.

One vial, confirmed medication coverage, and tons of pineapple cores later...

IUI Attempt #9: Unsuccessful

I wasn't surprised or disappointed. I owned my foolishness and hyper-optimism.

One more conversation coupled with Dr. S' recommendation, it was clear that IVF was my only option and I wasn't ready to own that. I took a break from my infertility journey.

Stats

ICI attempts = 2
IUI attempts = 9
Total Cost = $21950

Were you a recipient of the dye test? How did it go?

_____

_____

_____

*Did you use donor sperm or eggs? Did you learn
anything interesting about those options?*

_____

_____

_____

*How long did it take before IVF, if at
all, was your prescribed process?*

_____

_____

_____

Share your story at info@nashirabetton.com ♥

————— ✦✦✦✦✦✦ —————

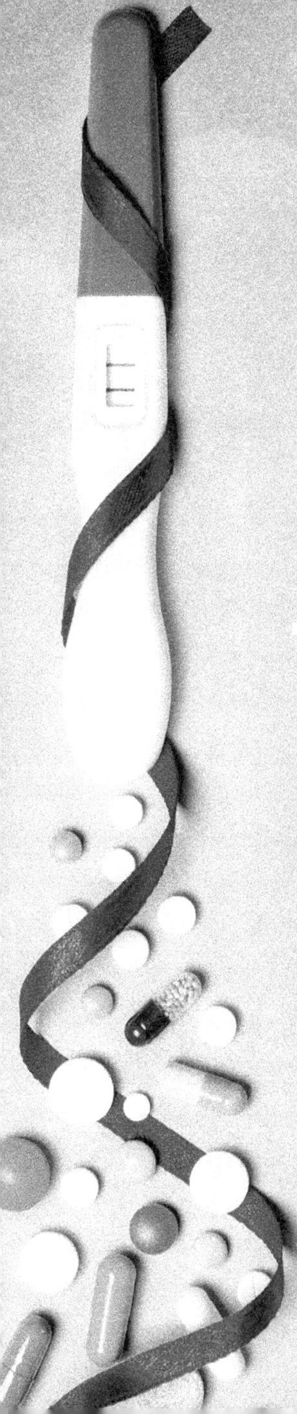

THIRD TRIMESTER

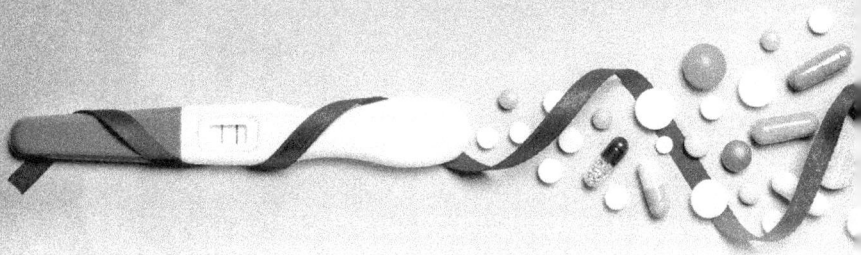

SHE DROPPED THE BOMB

For the next season, Summer 2014, I spent it focused on becoming a homeowner again. I figured that spending money renting wasn't ideal for me, especially if I had the moxie to pursue IVF in the future. I ended up landing a condo in an upscale area of Atlanta for a really great price. After enjoying my new home for a couple of months, the burning urge for a family reared its relentless head again.

In a more calm mental space and now riddled with the patience of a preschool teacher, because buying a home will force this on you whether you want it or not, I did my research in pursuit of a Reproductive practice near my new home in Atlanta. I read tons of reviews and researched each reproductive endocrinologist practicing at every viable facility.

To my surprise, I found a woman RE that looked like me! This was very important to me. It provided me with an inherent trust, although unfounded, because I felt she would have the compassion needed for this process and not simply take my money as I experienced before. This did make me partial, but it also created the confidence I needed to take a step in the needed direction.

I called the practice and set up a consultation appointment in August 2014. I approached this consultation much differently. I went in knowing I had to accept whatever was going to be my reality. Resisting fate would only prolong the outcome and let's just be frank, I had already spent 3 years trying and clearly I was doing it wrong, in many ways. It was time to cut the sh*t, buckle down, and listen to the fat lady sing.

One late summer morning, I was greeted by such a warm smile and pleasant voice from Dr. MK. It was at that moment that I knew I was "home" and boy was I right! Prior to this appointment, I had all of my previous doctors' files sent over and I even had the recordings, in hand, of my dye test. She was so well prepared for me. She had already reviewed every document and note in my files, viewed the images and videos of the dye test, and had a full explanation of her own analysis and recommendations. Super receptive, I hung onto her every word like it was gold nugget because, well, it was.

Her first recommendation was to complete a saline test[25], which is similar to the dye test but done in-house and with a sonogram. She wanted to verify with her own two eyes that the previous diagnosis was accurate and not a misfire. So that's what we did.

I was left in suspense for the remainder of the week as she compared her findings to those provided by previous

---

[25] Saline Test (Saline Infusion Sonohysterogram) - a procedure to evaluate the uterus and the shape of the uterine cavity. SHG uses ultrasound and sterile fluid to show the uterus and endometrial (uterine lining) cavity. The ovaries are also seen at the time of SHG. The purpose is to detect any abnormalities.

tests. On a Saturday afternoon I received a phone call from Dr. MK to discuss her final thoughts and recommendations. Talk about professionalism and quality service! Even on the weekends, she reaches out to her patients to ensure they are communicated to and in a timely fashion. I was surprised and nervous all at the same time.

She dropped the bomb. The IVF bomb. The bomb I wanted to avoid. The bomb I had to accept.

She confirmed what I already knew at this point. My fallopian tubes didn't effectively work and there wasn't a remedy for it, only a workaround. IVF was my workaround. I thanked her for her time and patience, and requested that she put me in contact with the IVF Financial Advisor. Within the next week, I had spoken with the advisor and understood exactly the cost, financing options, and processes to fulfill the monetary obligation.

Stats

Still…
ICI attempts = 2
IUI attempts = 9
Total Cost = $21950

What breaks from the process did you take and did it help?

_____

_____

_____

Have you experience a warm and fuzzy
feeling from your doctor? How was it?

_____

_____

_____

What financing options did you explore for your cycle(s)?

_____

_____

_____

Share your story at info@nashirabetton.com ♥

——— ·‧✦✦✦‧· ———

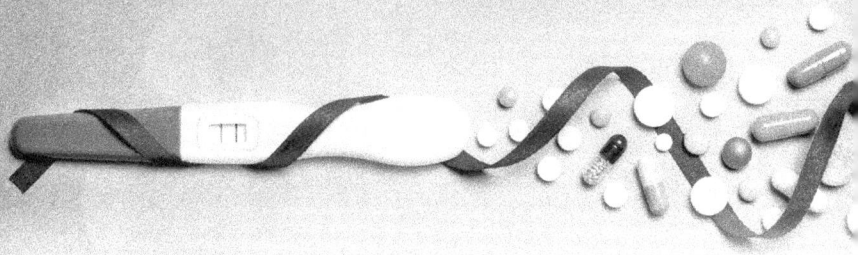

ELLEN, OPRAH

Even though I was a single woman embarking on this process, I made a decent salary, which disqualified me for any special programs geared to people in my situation. I looked for grants and other programs that would help offset the financial burden of this process. I quickly learned that unless I was a cancer patient or had some tear jerking story, I wasn't getting a damn penny. Although I wasn't part of those unfortunate circumstances, I applied anyway because nothing beats a failure but a try.

Needless to say, I didn't receive any assistance. So I tried the next best thing: sent emails to Ellen, Oprah, and every other notable television philanthropist. I thought my story to be unique enough to catch the eye of a woman who had loads of money and a heart to give. I never heard back from any of them *haha*. Can't say that was a total shocker but it was an itsy-bit deflating. My next course of action was what any resourceful person would do—crowdsourced funding. I created a profile on a popular crowdfunding website, wrote, then published my story, and set out on the pursuit to raise all the monies needed to get this process underway. I was sure I was going to hit jackpot with this approach, especially since I bared my soul and the "perks" you could receive were so freaking awesome. I mean who wouldn't want to be the recipient of:

- $25 – Creative Thank You Note: I will mail you a customized personal 'Thank You' note for your heartfelt contribution to my baby making journey.
- $50 – Say Cheese!: I will mail you a copy of Baby Betton's first ultrasound image + previous perks!
- $100 – A Lucky Charm: you will receive a custom bracelet designed for this cause by Lucky Charm Jewelry (view the Gallery for sample bracelets) + previous perks!
- $250 – Personalized Wreath: I will make and mail a customized wreath (view the Gallery for sample wreaths) for an occasion of your choice (holiday, birthday, etc.) + previous perks!
- $500 – Shhh! It's a secret!: You'll get first dibs on knowing the gender of Baby Betton in a very creative way + previous perks!
- $1,000 – Creative Baby Belly Cast: the thought of you being so generous warms me up with so much love that I will send you a creative cast of my baby belly + previous perks!
- $5,000 - Baby's Middle Name: yes, that's right! I will give Baby Betton your name as their middle name (or some derivative of it) + all the previous perks!

I was so grateful to receive lots of support from family, friends, and complete strangers who read my story. Although the money raised wasn't nearly what I needed to get started, it did help to pay for some diagnostic costs and doctor fees.

And just like that, I was back to the drawing board, again.

Stats

Still…
ICI attempts = 2
IUI attempts = 9
Total Cost = $21950

Were there programs you could apply for to acquire funding?

_____

_____

_____

Did you consider or use crowd sourced assistance?

_____

_____

_____

What ways did your family, friends, and/or strangers support your journey financially?

_____

_____

_____

Share your story at info@nashirabetton.com ♥

⸺⸺ ✦✦✦ ⸺⸺

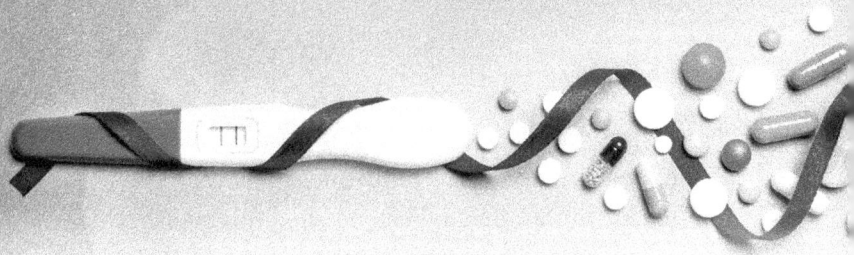

$1500 A MONTH

I'm sure I was not much of an anomaly with my financial state. I didn't have $20k sitting around waiting to be spent on IVF and I damn sure didn't have the additional $3k - $6k to spend on the medication or sperm. So I did what anyone would do with a hefty dream and determination—I financed it! If only it had really been that easy.

I applied to several (read: ALL) medical credit cards and loans. The problem with getting a medical loan is the challenging underwriting process—it is strict and unforgiving, which makes perfect sense. Here's why (amongst other reasons): when you finance a car or a house, you actually walk away with a vehicle or home as collateral. In the case you default, the said collateral can be seized or repossessed. Unlike cars and homes, getting a boob/nose job or having a baby doesn't leave the financing institution with something to relinquish, if the situation calls for it. As a result, their requirements are pretty stiff and interest rates higher than expected, no matter how great your credit is.

It's for this reason that I had a bit of a hard time getting a medical loan, and not to mention, I just bought a home months before impacting my buying power. I began applying for loans on a Monday morning and as quickly as the sun sets and rises, I had been denied by most lenders. Right before my eyes, I saw my dreams imploding fast. This was literally my last option before ending this quest became a true reality for the absolute last time.

I decided earlier on that I would practice patience this round so with 4 financers still pending, I held on tight to a small shred of hope. Wednesday and Thursday came then went; no news. On Friday, I heard from 3 medical loan companies, all willing to give me only a fraction of the cost. Can you say devastated?!

I guess this is where I should note the silver lining. When I added up all of the partial loans, together they equaled the total I needed. But they also, altogether, totaled more than $1500 in monthly payments for the next 4 years! The way the cost for childcare, diapers, clothes, and basic oxygen ranges for children, I just knew over $1500 a month wouldn't be conducive in the long run. Sure I *could* pay it but it just didn't seem like a smart plan. It was then that I accepted that I would have to terminate my journey.

My acceptance may have seemed premature or overly dramatic but what I failed to mention is: with every failed cycled and every cycle in between, I was still experiencing excruciating menstrual flows. My OB/GYN rendered me a candidate for a partial or full hysterectomy. This pain literally had a negative impact on my quality of life every 24 days. This meant that some months, I experienced the pain twice! For every month, a trying to conceive (TTC[26]) cycle was a bust or I wasn't able to try at all, I was pushed closer and closer toward the no baby zone.

---

[26] TTC - the time period in which they have intentionally been trying to have a baby.

As the day closed, I found myself entering into a state of depression. This was an all too familiar feeling of helplessness and defeat. I spent Friday evening, all day Saturday, all day Sunday, and all day Monday crying my poor little heart out. I didn't leave the house, I didn't eat, and I wasn't answering phone calls. I wanted nothing to do with the world or anyone in it. I went through this alone because alone felt better than everyone pitying me, or worse, me consoling everyone.

It was also during this time that I cursed God. I let Him have it! I couldn't understand how He could let someone able and willing go without the desires of their heart but then allow others who were unkind to their children, neglectful to their children, and flat out unloving to their children engage in parenthood. I was angry with Him and spent the entire weekend making sure He knew it.

I prayed to God that if I was meant to have the children I wanted, then He would have to make a way on the financial front. If He didn't then, I would accept my fate.

When I say God looks out for fools and babies, it's true, and this time, I was the fool.

Tuesday rolled around (Monday was a holiday), and I picked my fragile life together because duty called—my good ole 9-to-5. At some point during my work day, I received a phone call from a 1-800 phone number. Half listening, the woman on the other end identified herself as a representative for Medical Financing and called to let me know that I had been approved, but she needed more information before the loan could be processed.

I begrudgingly gave her the information she needed. At this point, I didn't really care that I was approved. I continued with the call just to be able to say I tried everything. Once she confirmed that I was absolutely approved, I then asked for the amount I would receive.

She responded. It was at this very moment that all feeling (and possibly blood *haha*) left my body. She had so sweetly stated that I had been approved for 100% of what I asked for and my monthly payments would only be $500!

Y'all I lost it!

I screamed in her ear as I shed tears of joy and I thanked her profusely. She was so happy that I was happy that she cried, too. I, then, had to double back to ask her to repeat her name and the company she called from since I hadn't truly listened in the beginning, and I wanted to be sure I said the right name in my prayers that night.

I remember that feeling like it was yesterday. I just knew with this victory, everything would fall perfectly in place and nothing could change my mind otherwise.

Stats

Still...
ICI attempts = 2
IUI attempts = 9
Total Cost = $21950

*Did you use a loan company? What medical
loan companies did you utilize?*

_____

_____

_____

How much money did you need from financing?

_____

_____

_____

*Did you ever share some choice words
with your Higher Power?*

_____

_____

_____

Share your story at info@nashirabetton.com ♥

•••♦♦♦•••

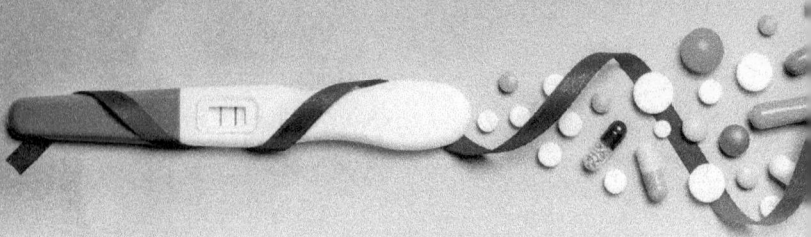

EASY BAKE OVEN

I secured the [money] bag!

By the beginning of September 2014, I had all the financial affairs taken care of for my first round of IVF. I also completed the authorization and ordering process, for the donor sperm, 4 weeks in advance to ensure that when the day comes to fertilize my eggs, there wouldn't be any problems. I did doubly confirm that my insurance did **not** cover any part of my IVF and I took it easy on the pineapple core as well *haha*.

Before the end of September, I had begun my fresh IVF cycle. I started on birth control then went through a series of blood draws to ensure that the recommended protocol was tailor made. To my surprise, the previous claims of diminishing ovarian reserve and quality, were not true. That behind me, I quickly ramped up to fertility meds once Aunt Flow reared her ugly head. I was on my medication protocol for nearly 3 weeks. During this time, I started to actually look pregnant, which was not a good thing. I swiftly learned what ovarian hyperstimulation syndrome (OHSS[27]) meant

---

[27] OHSS - the ovaries become dangerously enlarged with fluid. This fluid can leak into the belly and chest area, leading to complications.

and how it could negatively affect my cycle. Thank goodness it was a mild case but it was still a close call.

OHSS is simply when the hormones in the medication cause your ovaries to overstimulate leading to swelling and pain. In some cases, this swelling is so advanced that completing a fresh cycle isn't possible. The doctor will wait for your ovaries to return to its normal size before proceeding with an insemination. When this happens, the embryos are frozen until your body is ready resulting in a frozen embryo transfer (FET[28]).

I was so eager to get through this cycle, a frozen embryo transfer wasn't even on my radar and I had no interest in entertaining the thought of it.

By the time I finished my medication and was prepared for the egg retrieval process, I had grown 28 eggs. Secretly, I always felt like I had the potential to be Ms. Fertile Myrtle so I wasn't surprised by the high number at all J. The egg retrieval process was a breeze and I was grateful for it. I was even more grateful when my ovaries calmed down and returned to their normal size as their growth was quite uncomfortable.

Of the 28 retrieved eggs, 14 were considered viable. I thought to myself, could I possibly have 14 children, like in the olden days? Reality snapped me back swiftly when I thought about my current IVF payment plan and how 14 versions of any payment plan were enough to put my lavish dreams at bay. Of those 14 eggs, only 6 were able to be fertilized by my donor's sperm and considered sustainable for an actual baby by day 5 of incubation.

---

[28]   FET - referring to an IVF cycle using previously frozen embryos that have been thawed and then transferred.

On Friday, October 24th, my Easy Bake Oven of a uterus was inseminated with two great quality embryos. It was so surreal. It is STILL surreal. I couldn't believe that finally, FINALLY my uterus held what could be two future little me's! Look out world, here we come… or so I hoped!

This time, I wasn't going to deny myself the opportunity to be fully present with my two-week wait. See, before I waited a week and a half to test, if I even tested at all. This time, I told myself I was going to bask in every moment this cycle had to offer. This meant I was testing every single day starting the day after my insemination. I know, I know—I ran the risk of getting a false positive because of the fertility medication in my system but I didn't care. I was prepared to test the medication out until the test either remained white for a Big Fat Negative (BFN[29]) or faded out then faded in for a Big Fat Positive (BFP[30]).

Stats

ICI attempts = 2
IUI attempts = 9
IVF attempts = 1

---

[29] BFN (big fat negative) – negative pregnancy test.
[30] BFP (big fat positive) – positive pregnancy test.

Were there any complications or discomforts during your IVF cycle?

_____

_____

_____

Did you do a Fresh or Frozen cycle? Why?

_____

_____

_____

How many eggs were retrieved? Viable? Transferred?

_____

_____

_____

Share your story at info@nashirabetton.com ♥

———— ✦✦✦✦ ————

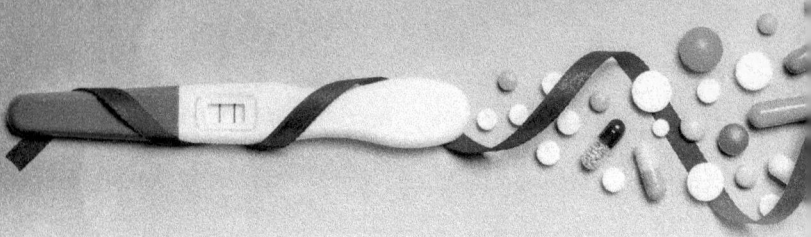

10 MORE DOLLARS

Prior to the transfer of my two beautiful embryos, I stocked up on dollar store pregnancy tests--roughly 10 of them! It may have seemed overboard, but I was in it to win it. Truly, they were only a dollar, and after having spent thousands of dollars on this process over the years, 10 more dollars wouldn't have tipped the scale.

With the first urine of every day[31], I tested:

1dp5dt	Positive (audible thought: likely false so I increased my water intake to flush out the trigger shot medication)
2dp5dt	Faint Positive (audible thought: likely still false so I drank water by the gallon)
3dp5dt	Clear Negative (audible thought: bummed because this could be the beginning of the end like before)

---

[31] First Urine – is the most appropriate specimen for pregnancy tests.

4dp5dt	Fainter Positive (audible thought: oh Lord the medication is still in my system *rolls eyes and chugs more water*)
5dp5dt	Faint Positive (audible thought: uhhhh, the medication should be gone by now *confused face and gulps more water*)
6dp5dt	Sort of Positive (audible thought: holy sh*t, this might have worked! *cautiously excited face*)
7dp5dt	BIG FAT POSITIVE!!! HAPPY F*CK*NG HALLOWEEN TO ME!!! (audible thought: please don't let this be an evil trick my body is playing on me!)

On Friday, October 31st, 2014, every tear cried, every surgery experienced, every dollar spent, and every prayer requested had finally been answered (I am in tears, right now, as I write this). At that very moment, my dream of motherhood came true. I worked so long and so hard, by myself, to be able to wear the honor of a mother, and it was slowly coming to life in my very own Easy Bake Oven. This experience of victory was PRICELESS!

Well, that's not *entirely* true—but, for those who like numbers, here it is:

Medication	x	~$5000*	=	$5000
9 IUIs	x	~$1500*	=	$13500
14 vials	x	~$650*	=	$9100
1 IVF	x	~$20000*	=	$20000
Total			=	$47600

*Calculated average or rounded cost

Ladies and Gentlemen…

On June 23rd, 2015 @ 5:34pm, I welcomed
to the world my darling son…

Micah Aidan Betton

The best gift life has ever given to me!

Stats

SUCCESS!

Did you test early during your two week wait?

_____

_____

_____

What were your overall/final infertility costs?

_____

_____

_____

How was the moment when you received your BFP?

_____

_____

_____

Share your story at info@nashirabetton.com ♥

————— ♦♦♦♦♦♦ —————

POST-PARTUM
CARE

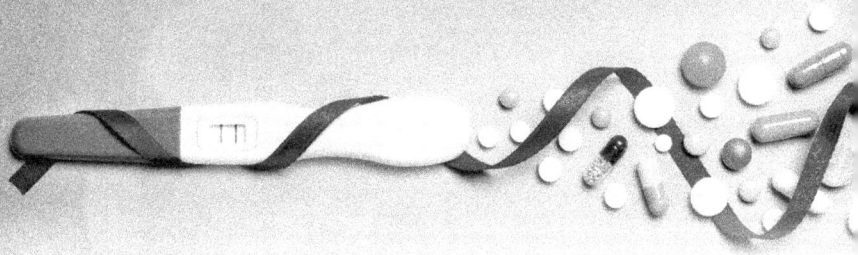

Delivery

I am humbled that you've taken time to read my story and have received a glimpse into my journey. I am even more humbled by your willingness to share yours. It takes courage and an insane amount of strength to relive a very trying experience that will one day help another in need. I honor you!

As I guided you through my journey, I asked thought-provoking questions with hopes to incite memories of the roads you once crossed. Those questions were only meant to scratch the surface. Please feel empowered to share as much or as little as you desire. There are so many topics not covered in my story and I would love to hear about all of them. This is your time to share the pieces that have created your path.

Outlined below are *"Fun Facts"* highly encouraged that you share. Feel free to remain anonymous and provide any important "facts" that are not mentioned. Once your story is written, please send it to ***info@nashirabetton.com,*** and it will be featured in an upcoming edition of the series. If you have any questions, feel free to send those to the same email address as well.

Fun Facts

First Name and Last Name Initial (optional)
City, State
Donor Egg (Y/N)?
Donor Sperm (Y/N)?
Cryobank Name (if applicable)?
Fertility Doctor & Practice (if applicable)?
Procedures Done (ICI, IUI, IVF), # of Attempts, # of Successes?
Number of Little Ones?
Cost?
Financing Used (if applicable)

Infertility is hard but not fulfilling life's dreams is even harder. Let's make this subject less of a taboo topic and one that encourages freedom and transparency. Your contribution will help to create a safe community for hope during this process. Much success on your family-building journey!

Stay encouraged. Stay uplifted. Stay strong.

Tell me your story...

_____
_____
_____
_____
_____
_____
_____
_____
_____
_____
_____
_____
_____
_____
_____
_____
_____
_____
_____

Glossary of Terms

Aunt Flow (AF) – popular euphemism referring to the menstrual cycle.

Anti-Mullerian Hormone (AMH) – protein hormone produced by special cells inside the ovarian follicles.

Big Fat Negative (BFN) – negative pregnancy test.

Big Fat Positive (BFP) – positive pregnancy test.

Clomid – ovulatory stimulating drug used to help women who have problems with ovulation.

Cytomegalovirus (CMV) – member of the herpes family of viruses that also includes chickenpox and mono.

Dye Test/Hysterosalpingogram (HSG) – involves placing an iodine-based dye through the cervix and taking x-rays to help evaluate the shape of the uterus and whether the fallopian tubes are blocked.

Estradiol (E2) – determines your ovaries' ability to produces eggs.

Ectopic – pregnancy that occurs in the fallopian tubes, when the tubes are blocked in some way, and the early embryo can't travel down to the uterus.

Egg Quality – refers to the state of an egg as genetically normal or abnormal.

Embryo – an unborn offspring in the process of development.

Endometriosis – condition where the lining of the uterus grows outside of the uterus. It is an abnormal and often painful disorder that affects anywhere from six to 10 percent of women.

Femara – fertility medication prescribed for women experiencing ovulation problems and/or unexplained infertility.

Frozen Embryo Transfer (FET) – IVF cycle using previously frozen embryos that have been thawed and then transferred.

Fibroids – noncancerous growths appearing in the uterus, usually during childbearing years, but they can occur at any age.

First Urine – most appropriate specimen for pregnancy tests.

Follicle Stimulating Hormone (FSH) – hormone that can directly influence your chances of conceiving and/or sustaining pregnancy.

Human Chorionic Gonadotropin (hCG) – hormone produced by the placenta after implantation and is detected in some pregnancy tests.

Intracervical Insemination (ICI) – involves placing sperm directly into the woman's reproductive tract to improve the chances of pregnancy.

Implantation –process of the egg burrowing into the uterine lining of the uterus.

Instagram – photo and video-sharing social networking service.

Intrauterine Insemination (IUI) – procedure involves transferring specially washed semen directly into the uterus via a thin catheter.

In Vitro Fertilization (IVF) – process of fertilization by extracting eggs, retrieving a sperm sample, and then manually combining an egg and sperm in a laboratory dish. The embryo(s) is then transferred to the uterus.

Laparoscopic – surgical procedure that involves making one, two, or three very small cuts in the abdomen, through which the doctor inserts a laparoscope and specialized surgical instruments.

Luteinizing Hormone Surge (LH) – triggers the start of ovulation, and the most fertile period of the menstrual cycle occurs.

Myomectomy – surgical procedure to remove uterine fibroids.

Ovarian Hyperstimulation Syndrome (OHSS) – when the ovaries become dangerously enlarged with fluid. This fluid can leak into the belly and chest area, leading to complications.

Saline Test/Saline Infusion Sonohysterogram (SHG) – procedure to evaluate the uterus and the shape of the uterine cavity via an ultrasound and sterile fluid to show the uterus and endometrial (uterine lining) cavity.

Trigger Shot – medication used after other fertility hormones to induce ovulation (release of the egg from the ovary) or to induce final maturation of the egg(s).

Trying To Conceive (TTC) – time period in which someone has intentionally been trying to have a baby.

Two-Wait Week - time it takes a fertilized egg implanted in the uterine wall to start emitting enough of the hCG hormone to be detected by a pregnancy test.

He has shown all you people what is good. And what does the LORD require of you? To act justly and to love mercy and to walk humbly with your God.
Micah 6:8

www.ingramcontent.com/pod-product-compliance
Lightning Source LLC
Chambersburg PA
CBHW022123280326
41933CB00007B/517